IS T
SICKNESS
OR AN
ENERGY
BLOCK?

KNOW THE DIFFERENCE
AND WHAT TO DO
ABOUT IT

AMY KEAST
INTUITIVE SOUL HEALER

ISBN: 978-19-5-036745-0

Published by

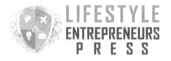

If you are interested in publishing through Lifestyle Entrepreneurs Press, write to: *Publishing@LifestyleEntrepreneursPress.com*

Publications or foreign rights acquisition of our catalog books. Learn More: *www.LifestyleEntrepreneursPress.com*

Printed in the USA

To my soul sister, Lily.
Thank you for never giving up on me.

Advance Praise

"If you have come across this book, there is a reason for it. The question will be, are you ready to find out what that reason is and be freed of whatever is causing your energy block? The healing will likely not be overnight, it will require work, and beyond work, it may also require you to set aside long-standing beliefs and coping mechanisms. This can be scary but in "Is This Sickness or an Energy Block? Know the Difference and What to do about it," the author, Amy Keast, Energy Healer, creates an accepting and raw environment, a metaphorical safe-space for the reader by sharing both her personal experiences and experiences of those that she has helped to heal. While she provides many valuable insights about the method of healing that resonates most deeply with her, she also acknowledges and touches on other methods the reader may explore along their healing journey. May this book encourage you to be brave enough to find the courage to follow your intuition to heal wholly and completely."

—Samantha Nowatzke, Regional Sales Manager,
Mutual of Omaha Insurance Company

"This was a highly interesting read and a beautiful dive into energy blocks, which blends the author's personal journey with informative teaching. I found the chapter on the original wounds fascinating; it helped me understand myself better. A lovely overview of this subject area and the author's work."

—Marianne Simpson, Writer

"I curled up on the sofa and dove into Amy's book. It flowed so well; I couldn't put it down. I will read it again. Though she takes you step by step through her healing journey, I can't imagine the challenges she encounters to uncover her truth. This story of personal growth is eye-opening and revolutionary. She explains various therapy options throughout the book, while encouraging you to find the right fit personally. I feel privileged to be a tiny step in the process. Thank you, Amy, for following your gut feeling, your intuition."

—Angie Kenkel, Mother of Five

"Not only is Amy an amazing healer, she provides an insight of various tools that one may use on their journey to emotional, spiritual and physical health. She explains basic ground level tools and creates an awareness of other modalities that may aid in your own healing process. Amy shares examples from her own life as well as others she has helped. This book is hard to put down once you begin."

—Elizabeth Book, Music Teacher

Contents

Foreword:

A Channel from Lily, My Spirit Guide

Thank you for allowing me to be heard and giving me a voice through you.

It is time in your world for change. Change in so many things, but for you, it's through healing that change has come and will come to others.

Healing energetically will become mainstream. Many will need to change their beliefs. This type of healing is not even possible for so many because of those beliefs. Many have prayed for such miracles, but when given the opportunity to heal, they won't believe it is possible.

Energy Healing will be considered the norm. New ideas are not always well-received or accepted. Healing once and for all will threaten many. Even those who are sick will battle with their own thoughts and feelings of becoming well. For so many, sickness is a way of life.

This is just the beginning of a massive shift in your society, of your culture looking outside yourselves in order to heal. Truly, healing starts within.

No longer will others be able to place the blame of sickness upon another or hide behind a diagnosis. Once the origins of sickness come forward, it's the dawn of a new era.

I'm excited to play a part in this change, this epic change. I wish I was in the physical world to do it alongside you as we had planned. I will continue guiding you as I have since your birth. We share a deep history together. The mission has not changed or my commitment to it. Together, we cannot be stopped.

We are not alone in this endeavor. There is a group of angels who surround you and protect you. Call upon them when you need them or don't feel safe.

I know we took the long route to get here, but there is nothing that can stop us now. All blocks have been removed and the path in front of you has been widened. So many opportunities await. You will be rewarded for your faithfulness.

Hang on. It's going to be a wild ride.

Your Soul Sister,
Lily

What You Can't See Can Hurt You

*"Change the way that you look at things and things
that you look at change."*

—Wayne Dyer

Throughout my life, I felt that something wasn't quite right, or that something didn't add up. There was a big question mark in the back of my mind. Was there something wrong with me? Was I sick? As a child, I experienced a great deal of sickness, all documented in my baby book. I was told that I had Celiac's disease and other ailments that sent me to the doctor and the hospital. Even after leaving home for college, I would find myself sick yet again upon returning home. I was also a sleepwalker. I often would go to sleep, then find myself in a different place when I woke up. Where was I going? Or, maybe I should have asked, "What was I running from?" The question mark for me was more internal, intuitive. I knew there was something that wasn't quite right, but I didn't put together what yet.

Being part of the medical profession for so many years taught me that when I feel sick, I don't want to run to the doctor. I don't need or want a pill to mask an ailment. However, I do want to do whatever I can to heal what I am feeling, especially if, God forbid, I really am sick. I'm going to do whatever it takes to have the best possible outcome. But, is this a sickness or an energy block?

You may come to me because you want the best possible outcome in order to heal. You want to take a bit of traditional medicine and mix it with the spiritual side, using what I have to offer to heal your current situation. You might realize that what you were doing was not working. You also realize that you want to get to the bottom of your sickness or energetic block. You are not sure what it is, but you do know that you need help.

What you do know is that this issue is causing you a lot of heartache. You would like to know or be able to decipher the difference between an actual sickness and an energy block, because knowing the difference would simplify your healing a great deal and allow for the best possible outcome. Not knowing keeps you in a state of confusion and doesn't allow you to heal.

Many of my clients come to me not knowing exactly what it is I do or am able to do for them. They are drawn to me somehow and are following their intuition. They know that there is a better way to heal, but they are not exactly sure what that is. Interestingly enough, many of my clients have energetic blocks that are similar to my own. I attract clients with the same type of wounds. (Surely, no accident.) Here's a list of other common traits many of my clients have.

They are:
- Intuitive.
- Current or former medical professionals.
- Dealing with mother issues.
- Dealing with abandonment issues.
- Lost because they didn't grow up in a nurturing environment for spiritual gifts.
- Under the belief that our current way of healing is outdated.
- Unsatisfied with their career or looking to transition to another.
- Dealing with childhood trauma.

As we get older, our bodies age, and many people think that these ailments we start experiencing are what is expected for our age. *Our bodies breaking down due to age* is a belief, and whatever you believe becomes your reality. An energy block turns into sickness when it reaches the physical body. Then, most people run to the doctor and the doctor tells them they have "XYZ." Patients leave the office happy to discover "XYZ," because at least now they know what they are dealing with. There's nothing that can be done to cure it; however, there is a pill that patients can take for the rest of their life that will manage their condition. But, taking it causes all sorts of side effects, causing the patient to need additional pills to combat the first pill. Our medical system is much more interested in naming a condition/illness/disease rather than curing it.

I think most would agree that our healthcare is really sick-care. We seek medical attention when there is a physical problem—when there is sickness. Working in the healthcare field for most of my adult life, I realize that we have it all wrong. We are managing symptoms rather than healing sickness.

It is possible to heal — we are simply going about it all wrong. We need to look inside and treat the soul. When the soul is healed, the physical body is able to heal. When there is a soul issue, the physical body responds with an illness.

The soul is energetic and has no physical form. We can't see it; it's deep inside. We are busy taking care of the outside, or the physical manifestations of our energetic block. We haven't paid attention to the subtle clues that are on the inside, screaming to get our attention. Ignored long enough, the blocked, stuck energy will turn into physical illness.

Intuitively, most of us already know this, but our society became ingrained in the system it created. What would happen if cancer was really cured? What would happen if there were no more diabetes or heart disease? What if people just dropped dead when it was time to leave this earth plane rather than after a long, debilitating sickness? A lot of people would be out of work. What would we do with all of those cancer centers?

What needs to happen is a change in the way in which we heal. We need to shift the paradigm and start healing on the inside. This step right now is completely ignored.

We could start by valuing our intuition and our spiritual gifts. That intuition is a valuable asset to every human being and the connection to their soul. This connection is the number one way to know that something needs to be healed, yet as a society, we don't value it. We should be teaching intuition development in our schools. Children are born wide open but begin to shut down their intuition when they begin their primary education.

As we get older, we lose connection with the soul. We ignore the messages it sends or simply quit hearing them. For me, when I got out of college, my soul cried out. I knew I chose the wrong profession but didn't know what to do about it.

Where have you lost your connection? What feels off for you? Are you busy looking everywhere else but within yourself for answers? It's a common mistake and ingrained in our society to seek answers outside ourselves. We're taught to want things and achieve certain goals, but what do you want? Do you even know? I went down this road before and completely understand how you must feel—lost and confused. As we travel down this road together, I'll share how I was able to reconnect with my soul. Certainly, you can do the same and find exactly what it is that you are looking for.

Hi, It's Me, Amy

"When it's all finished, you will discover it was never random."

—Anonymous

I grew up in a religious, conservative home. My parents were pillars of the community and the church. In my community, you were either Baptist or Catholic, and we were Baptist. Our home had a blue star in the window indicating it was a safe home for children if they needed it. My parents often took in young women who were in need of assistance and a place to stay.

Do you ever really know what is happening in someone's else home? I didn't see my father much as he was never at home. He would say that he was doing his job of providing. But, from the outside, one might ask, "Why doesn't he want to go home?"

When I was nine years old, my family moved from Omaha, Nebraska, to Harlan, Iowa. I don't remember almost anything prior to that move. I'm not sure why my parents picked Harlan, but it would be my home until I went to college.

There were lots of signs that something was not right, but I wasn't able to put that together as a child. My father was never home. I can count the times I saw my maternal grandparents on one hand. My parents didn't talk to each other and I never saw any affection between the two of them. I certainly received the message that they were not available emotionally. If I had a problem, I would not go to my parents for help. I didn't trust them. Something inside of me knew that they were not trustworthy. It was intuitive. I wasn't sure why others close to us didn't know that something was terribly wrong or chose to ignore it.

I didn't always know that I am intuitive. There were instances where I knew things without questioning how I knew them. The first time this happened was when I graduated from college and started working as a pharmacist. Almost immediately, I realized that I chose the wrong career. I didn't tell anyone; I thought there was something wrong with me. But I clearly received the message that I made a mistake. I felt it deep inside.

My father and his father were both pharmacists. I knew that both my parents would approve of my career choice. Pharmacy was a respected profession. So, I chose pharmacy in order to seek my parents' approval and because it was a safe choice.

When I realized I chose the wrong career, I wasn't sure what I should do. I just spent six years in college in a very selective field of education. I wasn't sure what to do with that. I made good money and that kept me at the pharmacy for the time being. I spent all of my spare time and money trying to figure out what I was feeling. I read books and went to self-help seminars, hoping to discover what appeared to be missing. Something inside me told me that I needed to find something else, that this wasn't who I was or what I should be doing. I considered going back to school for a nanosecond, but that didn't feel right either. I continued to search.

My intuition would reveal itself throughout my life. It was a voice I often heard. It was familiar and I trusted it. It was a part of me. I never questioned it.

> *Dream: I opened a cupboard and found a large bottle of vodka. The bottle was open. (A metaphor to opening the door to my spirit that was hidden away most of my life.)*

Like most kids in the public-school system, I took aptitude tests to see what type of career I would be best suited for. I don't think intuitive, psychic medium, or energy healer were part of that testing. I also didn't grow up in a home that embraced such things or valued spiritual gifts. I would have to go that path alone and figure it out for myself. Nobody talked about those things, or if they did, it wasn't in a positive way.

My healing work started to evolve when I recognized that people/society looks outside themselves in order to heal. Wouldn't it be great if every person knew how to look at their issues internally and decipher what energy block or issue they really had? I didn't have any idea what would transpire when I started energy healing. I just wanted to use my gifts and share them with other people. But I wasn't aware how to do that.

The beginning years of my work were mostly self-discovery about my spiritual gifts. By this time, I knew I was intuitive, and then realized that I was a medium and could channel spirits. Dreams were a way that I learned many things. The following dream I had back in 2012 about being a medium.

> *Dream: I went to the funeral home to pay my respects to a friend who recently died. The funeral director greeted me at the door. He escorted me to a room and said, "I think she is crying." I thought that was strange.*
>
> *I entered the room and my friend was sitting upright in the casket. She looked dead, but tears ran down her face. I asked her if she needed to talk and she nodded. I asked if she*

wanted me to give her husband a message. I knew what she wanted to say even though she couldn't speak it. I felt her emotion.

Working at the pharmacy turned out to be useful because it really helped shape my beliefs about our medical system. For the most part, our medical system is not working. It's not healthcare. It's sick-care. Why are so many people sick? Why are there so many cancer centers? Why don't people heal? These were the questions that I asked myself.

Our medical system is not all bad. The technology that is available to help people is incredible. But what really bothers me is the complete lack of responsibility that many have regarding their health. You only have one body. You need to take care of it. You don't need another pill.

What I'm going to be discussing about energy healing is not the norm; rather, it's a new thought that I am pioneering. I am sharing it so everyone has a chance to heal for themselves. I'll give you a peek behind the curtain about why it is that people don't heal. If this information challenges your beliefs, I suggest you check in with yourself and ask, "Is this belief mine or does it belong to someone else?" The next questions are, "What if I'm wrong? What is hanging on to this belief costing me?"

I discovered my healing gifts serendipitously. I didn't wake up one day and decide I wanted to be an energy healer. I didn't even know what that meant. I had no idea who I was or what my gifts were. It was like hide-and-go-seek, except I didn't know what I was looking for and I was blind-folded. This is because I have amnesia. I don't remember the first eight years of my life. All of the things that I know about myself were told to me. These are false memories because I don't remember any of them.

Spiritual Experiences

I'm no stranger to spiritual experiences. I had many throughout the years. Maybe you're not familiar with having spiritual experiences. I will share with you some of mine so that you may discover your own. Spirits are all around us and are seeking ways to communicate with you. Once they have your attention and make that connection, you will certainly have more.

A Phone Call from the Other Side

When my mother-in-law was dying, I sat by her bed and spoke to her. Our conversations were one-sided, and she didn't respond. A day or two before she passed, I asked her if she would give us a sign when she made it safely to the other side. I asked her if she would call and let the phone ring once. We would know it was her.

Following my mother-in-law's death, a week or two passed and my children would say, "Why hasn't Grandma called?" I wondered myself and worried that she may not.

It was a Monday evening. My husband was home for dinner and left to return to work. The phone rang and my youngest yelled that she would get it. I wasn't far and I could hear her saying, "Hello? Hello? Hello?"

By now, I was in the room with her asking her who it was. She proudly held the phone up high and yelled, "*It's Grandma!*"

Hearing Bells

Shortly before my mother-in-law's death, my sister-in-law and I both heard chimes like bells. It was like nothing I had ever heard before.

Seeing Spirits

I've seen spirits—not routinely, but on occasion when my youngest daughter was little. My daughter didn't like going to

11

bed or staying in bed. I would often sit downstairs in sight of her room to make sure she stayed in bed. One evening, after tucking her in several times, I saw what I thought was my daughter run around the corner of her room. I ran upstairs, hoping to catch her in the act, but what I found was my daughter fast asleep exactly where I left her with the door completely closed.

Touched by a Spirit

I've been touched several times, usually when I am sleeping, but there were other times as well. These experiences are a bit unnerving, and I came to realize that when a spirit is trying to get my attention, touching is good way to do it. There were a few times I was touched inappropriately. It all stopped when I realized who it was. In this instance, the spirit was my maternal grandfather wanting to give me his side of a story. He came to me another time to say that he was sorry.

My Mom Died Twice

The evening that my mother died, we all gathered around her. I sat near the top of the bed, stroking her eyebrows and talking quietly to her. I told her she could go. There was nothing left to do. We would be fine. I remember her taking her last breath, and I had a complete meltdown. Ten to fifteen minutes later, my mother took another breath and come back into her body. She seemed distraught, panicked, and not able to speak. She was no longer comfortable having me sit by her as I did previously. I was banished to the end of the bed. Why did she come back? Several hours later, my mother took her last breath for the second time.

Dream Visitation

My first dream visitation was from my mother shortly after she died. She appeared to me as a very beautiful, younger version of herself. She was all dressed in white. She stood before me, gripping her hands. I couldn't help noticing that she kept her head bowed and wouldn't look me in the eye. She told me she was getting better and would like to visit me on occasion, if that was fine with me. She also told me that this was her retribution. My mother continued to visit me in my dreams. It would take years for her to get down to business and tell me exactly what she meant by retribution.

Spirit Signs

Numbers, specifically repeating numbers (1111, 4444), are often used to get your attention from the spirit world. They are also referred to as angel numbers. Once you start noticing numerical patterns such as this, you will surely see more. You may notice these numbers on a clock or on a license plate. The numbers will pop up anywhere and help to remind you that you are a spiritual being. Numerical patterns such as these may help trigger/awaken your spiritual being. I experienced this often during my soul awakening.

Animals are also considered spirit signs. Each animal has their own meaning or significance. A sighting of a cardinal is believed to be a sign from a deceased loved one. I experienced this after my mother died. The cardinal would come around my home when our family would gather together. The bird would often peek inside the window. So, think of animals that appear randomly in your life. I often encounter the bat swooping in in the middle of the night. The bat is a symbol of death and rebirth, a sign of letting go of the past.

Dreaming is a high form of intuition. Each symbol is a message in itself. Once you learn your own dream style and how to interpret your dreams, the messages will increase and so will your connection to the spirit world. This is a perfect way to connect with your spirit guides.

Spirits don't talk to us in the same way we communicate with each other; spirits speak through symbols. They use numbers, animals, and music to express themselves. I often hear a song over and over again until I understand that it's a message that's just for me. Sometimes, I hear a song in my head. That song is the message. Music is one of my favorite spirit signs. I will often hear a song in my head. The song will keep playing until the message is understood.

When my childhood trauma resurfaced a while back, I heard the song, "Hold My Hand" by Jess Glynn. Why would someone want to hold my hand? I was being alerted. I was just about to be told something horrible. And so, my journey began.

My soul was urging me to remember who I am. In order to know/remember, I had to heal the deepest, darkest aspects of myself that were buried. I had a great deal of trauma in my childhood. I didn't remember any of it—there was a near death experience (NDE), massive child abuse, even electroconvulsive therapy (ECT). The ECT therapy may be the reason I have memory loss. I ignored those parts of myself that were not excepted or allowed. I completely separated from my true/authentic self. I took on behaviors, beliefs, and thoughts that would help me fit in with others and be accepted by the ones who mattered most: my parents.

I spent a great deal of time looking outside myself for the answers that eluded me. It wasn't until I started looking inside myself that the answers I sought appeared. It would be my intuition that guided me and would become my biggest ally, cheerleader, and friend.

I am an Intuitive Energy Healer and pharmacist. I'm married to my husband, Steve, and we have two beautiful daughters,

Madison and Ellen. We also have a fur baby, our dachshund Paul. I had a pretty normal life, or so I thought. I grew up in the Midwest, mostly Iowa. I did go away to college to Kansas University and spent the following six years in Arizona. I moved back to Iowa when I met my husband, and I've been there ever since.

My wish for you is that you will change the way you think and feel about sickness and disease. "You don't know, what you don't know." I'm here to share with you what you don't know so you can heal.

Why People Get Sick

"Truth passes through three stages:
First, it is ridiculed.
Second, it is violently opposed.
Third, it is accepted as self-evident."

– Arthur Schopenhauer

I took my professional knowledge from the physical world and meshed it with my knowledge of the spiritual world to share with you the truth about sickness and disease. The curtain that I'm pulling back for you will help you to discover a new way of healing and being. Healing truly is an inside job. We, as people and a society, need to learn to check in with ourselves rather than check out. When I say check in, I mean internally check in with your feelings and emotions. We are trained to look outside ourselves in order to heal. We have it all wrong.

It's important to know what an energy block is and how that relates to sickness. To help clarify, I'll share with you what I've learned as a healer.

First, healing isn't always a quick process. Peeling back the layers of trauma often takes time—time to discover, time to process, time to heal. The layers I speak of are that of the different energetic fields that need to be cleared: the mental field, the emotional field, and the soul field.

The traumas that need to be processed are typically experiences from childhood through your late twenties. These events are things you were not able to process because your brain was not fully developed. As children, our brains are not able to process trauma, so it sits in various energetic fields, our energetic bodies and minds, waiting to come out and be healed. To complicate things further, you probably won't remember this trauma as the mind does an excellent job of hiding it to keep you safe.

I'll take you through the chakras to discover the types of energetic blocks that can be stuck there, and I will give you examples of the types of illness that occur when a block is present in that area.

Together, we will peel back the layers of healing. I'll share with you some of my healing and some of my healing work as well.

Intuitive healing is my specialty, but it's not the only way to clear stuck energy. You'll learn that there is more than one way to heal. You can heal yourself, you can seek assistance, or you can do a combination of the two. When you need help, ask for it and seek it out. I'll give you those tools.

One of those tools that works best for trauma is eye movement desensitization and reprocessing (EMDR) therapy. Hypnosis is another great tool. These are effective and easy to use. What I will be discussing in this book are what tools I used and how I personally healed.

Next, we will discuss the various forms of stuck energy, or the negative energy that becomes stuck in our energetic bodies. This energy gets stuck because it has a low vibration—think of it as being sticky. These lower vibrational energetic blocks are past life issues, negative feelings, false beliefs, negative emotions, and trauma that hasn't healed.

I'll share with you the ways of clearing stuck energy/energetic blocks. Some of these ways to clear your energy can be done

17

independently, while others may require assistance. I'm sharing with you all of the nuggets of information that I used to heal. I'll throw in a few of my experiences to help you with yours.

We will also discuss the big question: How do I know if I have stuck energy? You will learn the tell-tale signs of stuck energy and how it appears in your life. We will discuss the emotions to look for, the patterns that appear, the triggers, and what it all means.

I will also introduce you to the soul chakra, often called the zero chakra. This is the place where real physical change will occur when healed. The soul chakra is the chakra that was neglected in healing our true self. Everything starts at the soul level.

After the soul chakra, we will discuss the original wound. Finding the original wound is critical if you want to heal once and for all. The original wound is always attached to the soul, and I visualize this as a root that needs to be pulled out. Skipping this step is the reason people don't heal. We will discuss why our current medical system is failing us, and I'll give you examples of the original wound.

In addition, I'll explain my intuition and my spiritual gifts and how they work. I will also introduce you to the voice of my intuition and how that came to be.

My work and my life are what some would call "stranger than fiction." In order to become who I am today, I had to shed who I was told to be. I had to discover my original wound and heal my soul. It wasn't easy. I lost a few people along the way. Time does not heal all wounds; it buries them.

Energy Healing

"The light in me honors the light in you."

– Anonymous

Energy Healing Types

Energy Healing is the science of releasing stuck energy in the body, whether it be physical, mental, emotional, or soul-related. There are many types of energy healing—Chios, Reiki, the Clearing Statement, tapping (EFT). Intuitive Energy Healing is my specialty, but before developing my own method, I was learning everyone else's.

Chios is a very extensive and complicated channeling of universal energy. This method can be used in-person or through distanced healing sessions. This is a deep-dive type of learning and may take years to fully understand. If you're interested in certifications regarding energy healing, this is what you are looking for. I used this educate myself about channeling and the modality of energy healing.

Reiki, another channeling of universal energy, was developed over one hundred years ago by Mikao Usui. At that time, and for the next hundred years, Reiki was revolutionary and ahead of its time. This type of energy healing is considered a hands-on method. You'll often find that Reiki is used during massages, acupressure, and is excellent for animals.

The Clearing Statement comes from Access Consciousness and consists of a bunch of words that are used to bypass the logical mind in order to clear stuck energy. The Clearing Statement is, "Right and Wrong, Good and Bad, POD and POC, all nine, shorts, boys, and beyonds." You might find yourself using The Clearing Statement for thoughts and beliefs that you wanting to eliminate.

Tapping, or EFT, is one of the first methods that I utilized and still do today. This is a system where you tap on various meridian points on your body, as in acupressure, in order to release stuck energy. EFT, which stands for emotional freedom technique, was created by Gary Craig. Tapping is great for anxiety, fears, smoking cessation, and anytime you find yourself aware of an issue that is preventing you from moving forward.

Intuitive Energy Healing

My work is intuitive. I utilize my intuition in order to recognize what needs to be healed. I identify the stuck energy. The healing occurs simultaneously as I channel spirit energy to clear the stuck energy. This is a frequency that releases the negative energy. It is a gift that I have.

Everything is energy. In my energy work, it's the negative energy that causes the problems. Negative energy vibrates at a much lower frequency and becomes stuck in various energy fields. The energy fields that I work with are the mental, emotional, physical, and the soul-related fields.

I didn't always know that I am able to do this, and nobody trained me. I didn't learn in a seminar or in a self-help book. I learned this skill the hard way—by working with other people and through my own healing. It wasn't a fast or easy process, but what I learned will change the way we think about sickness and disease.

My intuition was always present, but it was not something I acknowledged or talked about with others. It was taboo—at least in my home. As I grew older and had a family of my own, my intuition became more pronounced and something I became interested in. Again, I didn't fully acknowledge or talk to others about it, but as I became more interested in my own intuition, my intuition expanded.

I began to wake up spiritually during my dream time. Dreaming is considered a high form of intuition and an easy way to connect with the spirit world. Dreaming was the beginning of my self-discovery and the path to learn about my spiritual gifts. However, first I had to learn what the dreams meant, as well as what type or style of a dream I was having. Dreams are rarely literal. In fact, each symbol in the dream represents a message. Spirits don't communicate as we do in the physical world, but they will communicate through symbols and spirit signs. When you find a way of communicating effectively, such as dreams, the conversations you have will escalate. My dreams were how my spirit guide would speak to me. If I didn't understand the dream, or I had the wrong interpretation, the dream would repeat.

In 2011, after my mother died, she started visiting me in my dreams. I uncovered more spiritual gifts with the discovery of channeling spirit energy and mediumship. It was an interesting time, and I had much to learn.

I journaled these experiences and started a blog. I discovered that there were a lot of people just like me who were interested in the spirit world but were not comfortable talking about it in public. I shared what was happening with me and thought it might help others.

I started giving readings in exchange for feedback. The feedback that I received was not what I was expecting. People would tell me the reading was fine, but something else happened to them during the reading that they couldn't explain. Somehow, they were feeling lighter emotionally, or an obstacle was cleared for them.

I didn't understand at first, but soon gained that clarity by using my intuition. I realized that something was being cleared when I performed readings for people, so I started to use my intuition to identify what I was clearing. This was the start of my conscious intuitive energy healing. I say "conscious" because up until that point, the clearing was completely unconscious to me and the people I worked with.

I attracted people who have issues alarmingly similar to my own—no mistake there. This was always an opportunity for some healing of my own. I often wondered why I couldn't simply clear my energy once and for all and get on with it, but it didn't work that way. I had to peel back every layer. It would take years to heal and fully understand each and every issue I had.

For example, if you and I were sitting down in a session, how this works is that I would feel into your energy. Often times, it feels like someone threw a blanket over me. That blanket is emotions that I sift through. It's the emotions that tell me a story, your story. As I identify the negative or stuck energy, magically it is cleared. The channeling of energy is a frequency that disrupts the holding pattern in the energetic field. It sounds fancy, but it is simple.

What Does Intuitive Energy Healing Look Like for You?

If you were my client, we would meet either in person, via video chat, or on the telephone—our meeting doesn't need to be physically in person. We are all connected and energy flows to where the intention is set. I would energetically connect to you through your heart chakra. This works in a group setting as well.

I prefer that you don't give me any information prior to our connection. Rather, I like to tell you how the session will go and then we have a conversation about what I am feeling or sensing about you. I typically work from the bottom chakra to the top and from the outside in. This is how my work was for years, but there was something that didn't seem right. I wondered: Why were my clients coming back to me? Didn't I do the job right? Wasn't the healing one and done? I felt as if I wasn't doing something right or was something missing. I realized what was happening here was that I was peeling back the layers. I was clearing their obstacles one at a time, much like I was doing for myself.

I was clearing the emotional and mental bodies. These were the things that, if left un-cleared, would turn into a physical illness. I was finding vows from past life experiences. I was also discovering soul issues from past lives that somehow became activated in this lifetime. I continued to help those that came to me and I healed myself day-by-day.

I use my spiritual gifts in my sessions with others. I am a medium and receive guidance from my spirit guide. That information comes to me in various forms: I either hear it, see it, feel it or just know. It's that simple.

In my own healing came new discoveries. The soul itself is where healing needs to take place, because this is the place of the original wound (the place where all the trauma starts). All of the remaining trauma and emotional and mental pain are stacked upon each other, layer-by-layer. Think of it as peeling an onion in reverse; you're adding layers rather than taking off. Another way of thinking about it would be to visualize bricks, or a foundation in which bricks are stacked. There's the foundation of the trauma and then the incidents in life that stack up against the foundation. This would be what turned my work upside down. I was working from the outside-in, but what I should have been doing was going straight to the soul and disrupting the foundation. Without a proper foundation, the rest of the bricks don't stand a chance. I didn't realize any of this until my own soul was healed. That's when the truth hit me, and my work completely changed. I went straight to the soul.

A soul healing addresses the issues of the original wound—that first wound in the current lifetime that deeply hurt you. The original wound is often encompassing beliefs such as, "I'm not lovable," or, "I'm not enough." It can also be a trauma. It is the culmination of thoughts, feelings, and beliefs that were not processed.

I had a great deal of trauma in my childhood, none of which I remember. I have a condition called retrograde amnesia, and I have no conscious memories of the first eight years of my life. I had an NDE (near death experience) that would change my life forever. Everything prior to that experience is wiped from my memory. I didn't get those memories back. I do know about my life because I have a spirit guide who told me, and I did much healing work around that. For years, I thought that these missing memories were the reason my work was not yet complete. It wasn't this trauma, but the original wound that needed to be healed. My trauma occurred in-utero, shortly after conception.

I've seen this happen before because I had lots of clients with issues in-utero, typically because a pregnancy was unwanted or unplanned. How this manifested for my clients was that, although they may have not known anything about an unwanted or unplanned pregnancy, they did know how they felt—unloved, unwanted, or not enough. They also would spend most of their life seeking that approval from their parents. This feeling of not being loved or wanted was the underlying issue is their lives.

Healing the soul is the key to healing, period. People don't have to heal layer upon layer in order to finally get to their original wound. Certainly, you heard of individuals who were in therapy their entire life. Despite all of their counseling, many people did not find the original wound, which needs to be healed. Not all original wounds start in-utero, but you can see that if they do, it will take a long time to figure these issues out because people aren't looking there or considering trauma that occurs before their birth.

In our modern healthcare system, we are not treating the whole person—we are only treating the physical body. Throughout my pharmaceutical career, I learned that most people don't get better; they get another pill. Drugs are not always the answer. We need to start asking better questions in order to change how we heal. Why are there so many cancer hospitals? If someone's cancer went into remission six months ago, why does it come back now? Disease returns because we don't find the cause, or in this case, the original wound.

The Traditional Chakras

*"If we worked on the assumptions that
what is accepted as true really is true,
then there would be little hope for advance."*

– Orville Wright

The chakras are the invisible energy centers located from the bottom of your spine to the crown of your head. They are invisible to the naked eye; I don't see them, but I do perceive them. I know that some people do see them, but most do not. For this discussion, I am only talking about the main chakras that line up with the physical body. There are other chakras, but we aren't going to discuss those here. For years, my work consisted of working with only these chakras. I'll share with you some of the issues I discovered.

The Root Chakra

The root chakra is at the base of the spine and is the energetic field that connects us to the earth. This is the field where I find issues with stability, safety, or basic human need issues. The root chakra is where you store your beliefs, or the information that you pick up from your parents. In their early years, children are like sponges and soak up literally everything that is around them. Around the age of nine, the brain forms a partition separating the conscious and the subconscious minds. Until then, the information coming into the brain flows directly into the subconscious. The first eight years of a child's life are very important for stability and feelings of safety. You can see how this might be a problem as we grow older. You may not remember something from your childhood, as your mind tries to keep you safe, but the feeling of being unsafe is stored in your subconscious and it may be an underlying issue in your life.

The bones and the skeletal structure correlate to this chakra. If you have an issue with your bones, such as arthritis, then this is a root chakra issue.

As I mentioned before, beliefs are also stored in the root chakra. One hundred percent of your beliefs are taken from your parents, or whoever is raising you. As we get older, most of us start to recognize that not all of our parents' beliefs are our own, and we start to form new beliefs based on our own reality. Once again, these beliefs are stored in the subconscious mind. Not all beliefs are good or bad. The beliefs that I see in my work are beliefs with a lower negative vibration, such as, "I'm not good enough," "I'm not lovable," or, "I need to be perfect, or they won't love me."

The Sacral Chakra

The sacral chakra is the source of sensuality and creativity. This is also the energetic connection to money and where the connection to the emotional body resides.

I often see victimization here, typically sexual in nature. If you took a vow of celibacy, or a vow of poverty, I would see that here as well. Vows are typically a past life issue—something you agreed to in another life. I'm certain most wouldn't agree to such vows today, unless you were a priest or nun, and I cleared that issue for so many people.

This is also where womb and fertility issues manifest as well. Ladies experiencing issues with fertility, menstrual cycles, or the womb are all experiencing issues somehow related to their mother.

Money is an energy, and often people get hung up on working hard and have certain beliefs around their money. All of those things interfere with the energy of money. I heard back from many clients who told me that almost immediately following our session, they asked for a raise and received well over what they expected. I also had clients who were promoted or changed to a job more suited to them.

Meet Jamie

Jamie came to me after she'd suffered her most recent miscarriage, the latest of many other previous miscarriages. She was experiencing fertility issues and suffering multiple side effects. She was seeing a specialist, but still having all sorts of difficulties of the female kind.

What I discovered with Jamie was she was abandoned from her mother in a previous lifetime, but the mother kept her sister.

This is what I would call a soul issue. My client didn't recall this, but her soul remembered the experience.

In Jamie's current life, her mother was very loving and did not abandon her. However, Jamie's sister was having a personal struggle of her own and for a time needed to move back home with her parents. To Jamie, her mother chose her sister over her all over again. The soul issue was causing her fertility issues, and on a personal level caused her heartache with her mom and sister. Her feelings were real, but on a conscious level she never fully understood why she felt the way that she did. The feeling of abandonment is a heart chakra issue, while the issues of the womb are related to the sacral chakra.

Meet Lucy

I met Lucy in a group energy session. During this group session, I went through the chakras as I normally do. When I got to the sacral chakra, I heard the words, "We can't talk about it." I felt grief and loss. This did not resonate with anyone in the group. I skipped over this chakra and said that we would come back to it. Going back to that energy, I heard it again—"We're not supposed to talk about it." Still, no one spoke up. I asked the ladies if they wanted me to move on. No, they all agreed that they wanted to heal the issue that was coming up. I then heard, "People don't talk about these things and be grateful for what you have." Lucy now spoke up and said that she had twins and one of them died at birth 40 years ago. She was told that she should never talk about it. They had a healthy baby. They should be grateful for what they have. The pain that was buried for so many years was coming up to be healed. Lucy told me that she had female medical issues ever since.

Again, most often when I see a woman with fertility issues, menstrual cycle issues, or womb issues, she is experiencing problems with her mother.

The Solar Plexus

The solar plexus is your power center, the ego center, and your perception of who you are. This is your self-esteem, discipline, and your warmth of personality.

This center is related to the endocrine system. Blocks in this area result in loss of power and loss in self-esteem.

As a child, I wasn't allowed to be myself. My mother didn't want me and did not approve of my spiritual gifts. This diminished my self-worth and gave me a false perception of who I am. I had a massive block in my solar plexus—my power center.

Healing the solar plexus involved discovering who I really am and allowing that little girl to heal—more peeling back of the layers.

Meet Stella

I met Stella as she was waking up spiritually in mid-life. She spent most of her life taking care of everybody else while neglecting herself in the process. She was just uncovering her soul and beginning to find herself when we worked together. I found that at a very early age, Stella lost her childhood. She was expected to take care of her siblings, cook, and clean the house. She lost her power. More specifically, her power was stolen from her. She was victimized and not allowed to speak of it. She was made to believe that it was her fault and was shamed for that. Her childhood trauma was never processed or allowed to heal.

The Heart Chakra

The heart chakra is all about love—being loved, feeling loved. The pains and the abuses of those feelings are stored here. I often see patterns with the heart chakra, in that it is often directly related to other chakra issues (i.e. a person who was victimized would have a block in their heart chakra as well). A person who believed they were not lovable would have a heart block in addition to the root chakra issue. You can see how these issues start to pile on top of each other and in layers.

The Throat Chakra

The throat chakra is your voice and involves speaking your truth. Shame blocks this chakra and is also present with multiple chakra blocks, just as the heart is. If you have a blocked throat chakra, you would most likely see a thyroid problem or difficulty speaking your truth.

The throat chakra is often blocked whenever there is any type of trauma. Children are often told not to speak of an abuse or trauma. It's not the actual silencing of that trauma, but the shame that is placed around it. Stella had a blocked throat chakra from her victimization in childhood.

When I am doing an energy clearing, I see shame as hands around the throat, as if someone is being choked. I might also cough or the person I'm working with may cough. These are all signs that the throat chakra is blocked.

The Third Eye

The Third Eye is the gateway to higher consciousness—it's your intuition in all forms and it's your inner voice and internal GPS. Everybody has intuition, but the problem is that we don't always listen to it. If you want your intuition to expand and grow, pay attention to it. Intuition is key in my work and in my life. If I did not listen to my intuition over the years, I would have nothing. Blocks in this area could be present themselves as a disconnection from intuition or as sinus problems and eye problems.

The third eye is where all of the "clairs" reside: clairsentience, clairvoyance, clairaudience, Clair cognizance, Clair olfaction, as well as empathy.

Clairsentience means clear feeling, while clairvoyance is defined by seeing clearly through visions. Clairaudience is the ability to hear spirits, which most commonly present itself as clear thoughts, and Clair cognizance is knowing things without reason. Finally, Clair olfaction is the gift of psychic smell. Psychic smell is smelling a loved one's perfume or cigar. It's that smell that instantly connects you to that person. Psychic smell is also considered a spirit sign.

I developed most of those, but I would say that being empathic is what defines my intuition most. Empathy is feeling the emotions of others. As an empath feels the emotions, their mind goes to work to decipher the meaning of those emotions.

The Crown Chakra

The crown chakra is our connection to the universe and the life force through the other six chakras.

This chakra corresponds to the conscious and the subconscious mind. Someone with multiple sclerosis, Parkinson's, Alzheimer's, or who suffers from migraines or other neurological disorders have a block in the crown chakra.

Since the crown corresponds with the mind, conscious, and the subconscious, I often find this to be one of the most fascinating chakras. It is helpful to know that your mind is always trying to keep you safe. You may not remember your trauma because the brain is doing its job. That's a coping mechanism of the mind.

For those people with Alzheimer's and dementia, they are trying to forget. It is something that is so painful that their mind erases it. It's trauma.

To sum things up, specific diseases and health conditions correlate to specific chakras. Knowing which chakra is affected will help you discover what exactly is stuck in energetically in your body. Start thinking of stuck energy in your body as something that needs to be removed rather than something taking up permanent residency.

What Causes Stuck Energy

*"You can never change things by fighting
the existing reality. To change something,
build a new model that makes
the existing model obsolete."*

– Buckminster Fuller

What exactly is the cause of stuck energy? As you continue reading, keep in mind that I use the words "block" and "stuck energy" synonymously.

As we discussed earlier, children are not able to process trauma or negative energy, so anything of a negative nature/ frequency gets stuck in a child's energy field due to the fact that, until a child is nine years old, the partition between the conscious and the subconscious mind is not formed. It was also proven that, up until a person's late twenties, the brain is not fully developed. Indeed, this information correlates with what I am finding in my work, as it is not only children who are not able to process trauma, it's young adults as well.

What constitutes trauma is anything that a child perceives as negative. It may not be negative, but the child interprets it as negative or a lower vibration. Remember, a child's undeveloped brain does not process trauma, so these experiences are stored in the subconscious and the appropriate chakras. The essence of this is how something makes you feel. There may be no words or conscious memory, but rather a feeling that persists.

A death in the family is trauma. The loss of a pet is trauma. A car accident is trauma. All of these things are trauma, but may not necessarily cause stuck energy. It's the thoughts, feelings, and beliefs that go along with the trauma that cause the problem. It's the stories we tell ourselves regarding the trauma. None of the stories that you are telling yourself may be true, but after a while, those feelings turn into beliefs. This is when the energy become stuck or blocked.

Meet Mary

Mary was adopted. She didn't care that she was adopted and had no intention of ever meeting her birth parents. But, when her adoptive parents passed away, she started having some health issues. She had random thoughts of her husband leaving her. She worried her children would move away and she would be all alone.

Now mind you, Mary is a very successful woman who had a brilliant career and loving family. Her anxiety stemmed from an abandonment issue. She worked on herself over the years through personal development and was perfectly happy that she was adopted. She was raised in a loving home and had a wonderful family. She didn't give her adoption a second thought in years.

The issue arose when her adoptive parents died, and the unhealed wound of abandonment was reignited. Her fears became her thoughts and anxiety took over. This is the time in life where most people run to the doctor for a pill to mask those feelings, because, plain and simple, this hurt does not feel good. Others self-medicate with alcohol or drugs. However, this is the time to ask yourself what is really going on and to seek out some help.

Anxiety is a symptom of something deeper that wants to be healed. There isn't a drug for that. You have to feel it in order to heal it, or to find yourself someone like me to identify and clear it with you.

Meet Luke

I met Luke at a seminar a few years back. He was a young man and I was surprised to learn that he had multiple sclerosis (MS). I told him about my energy work and asked if I could give him a session in exchange for feedback.

I wasn't prepared for what I learned. I found it shocking.

Luke had a past life issue or soul issue of torture. Something in this lifetime triggered that memory in his soul. The trigger was extreme parental control. Luke was not able to be himself because he was being controlled. Luke went on to tell me how controlling his parents were while he was growing up. They chose his career and college without regard for his desire. He also told me that he had three recurring dreams where he was being tortured.

Today, Luke is living his dream, not his parents' dream, and he no longer has torturous dreams.

Past life issues are stuck energy from another lifetime that the soul wants to heal. Trauma that was not healed will be buried. There will be no signs of this. In fact, you may not even be aware that you are burying your trauma because your mind is doing a terrific job of keeping you safe. For example, I didn't know I had trauma in my childhood. The amnesia took care of that. The unhealed trauma will present itself when the soul feels that it is safe to do so.

A few months before my mother passed, it was obvious that she didn't have much time left. I didn't have a great relationship with my mother, and I realized that if I wanted answers from her, I needed to get them while I could. I didn't like my mother and she didn't like me. I didn't know why, and I was always afraid to ask. When I finally began asking the hard questions, I received no response. My mother wasn't talking. She literally took her feelings to the grave.

When my mother took her last breath, I had a gut-wrenching breakdown. My body shook all over and something deep inside of me cried out. It was my soul and she was ready to heal. Finally, it was safe to come out. That was just the beginning of my healing and it would take me years to get through the layers upon layers of stuck energy.

If I did not allow myself this time to heal, who knows what would have happened to me? Who knows what sicknesses I would have developed?

What I do know is that my healing was all-purposeful and that each person who came to me was showing me something I needed to heal within myself. They were my mirrors. Their energetic blocks were my mine. I was attracting people into my life who were just like me. People who needed to heal what I needed to be healed.

The Split

While working with others, I discovered an unusual finding of what I call, "the split." I found that not only is trauma that happens to us is a cause of stuck energy, but so is the trauma that we do to ourselves. We have a relationship with our self, our soul. There are times when we turn against or reject who we are. It's a survival mechanism. The soul breaks or splits in order to separate from a feeling or belief. This energetic split is where another layer of sickness and disease originates.

I had my own splits to heal. I wasn't loved for who I was, so I opted to forget and rejected those parts of myself that were deemed unworthy. I created a split in order to eliminate the heart ache of not feeling loved.

A split is where a person energetically turns off the lights or the flow of energy in our own soul. When you turn off the lights, and never go into that space again, that split fragments from the soul. It's self-preservation pure and simple.

Meet Sharon

Sharon is a fifty something, business professional with a very busy lifestyle. She is recently seeing a doctor for extreme fatigue and other hormonal related issues. As I tuned into Sharon, I find a victimization wound from an early childhood age that Sharon knows nothing about. She has no recollection, no nightmares, but she does feel as if her memory is fading. Sharon asks if I can tune into her mother as well.

Meet Anne

Anne has full-on Alzheimer's and is living in a care facility. Ann's energy strangely enough had a wound similar to Sharon's. While Sharon was the victim, Ann had the knowledge and kept it a secret. Where Sharon didn't remember, Ann tried to forget.

It became clear to me that it wasn't just the trauma that they had experienced causing their physical problems. Each of these ladies both turned on themselves in some way. They rejected a part of themselves in order to distance themselves from the emotional pain they were feeling. It is this split within themselves that causes the memory issues, the Alzheimer's.

Wondering if you have energetic blocks? If you have a chronic illness/disease, then I can tell you with one hundred percent certainty that you have an energetic block.

Ways to Clear Stuck Energy

*"Open your mind and clear it of all thoughts
that would deceive."*

– Ralph Waldo Emerson

When my kids were both in elementary school, I started thinking about my career once again. I wanted something more, but still didn't know exactly what that looked like. I stumbled across hypnosis training and I thought that would mesh with my pharmacy career. I was excited to learn something new.

I attended the weekend seminar with a few hundred others, many of whom were already trained and practicing hypnosis. This training was my introduction to regression hypnosis, which occurs when you take a person back in time through hypnosis. The host of the seminar often brought up regression, but did not want to talk about it and refused to take questions concerning regression. Regression was not discussed at the seminar, but was instead the side conversation throughout the breaks and downtime. What I was hearing was that not only did regression work in taking a person back to another time in their life, but you could also regress a person back to another lifetime.

My mind almost exploded. Why didn't I know this? Why didn't people talk about things like this? And then I learned why. This did not line up with a lot of people's beliefs or their religion. I needed more information to decide my opinion on regression. This was ground zero of my healing work. For a time, I did hypnotize people mostly for smoking cessation and a few other health-related issues. Hypnosis wasn't my favorite energy healing practice, but I learned some amazing things about the mind and, of course, about past life regression. This would all be very helpful to me one day.

I started using hypnosis for myself in my personal development work. I worked with Marisa Peer in a seminar and a home study course, and I found it incredibly healing. Marisa uses a style of hypnosis called Rapid Transformation Therapy (RTT) and trains others in this practice as well. Hypnosis was important in the development of my work and critical in my healing.

I learned a great deal about both the conscious and subconscious mind during my hypnosis training and healing. In my own sessions, I was taken back to a time in my life where healing needed to be done. I didn't have to recall the incident. My mind was just instructed to go there and release the trauma. I was then given new instructions in place of the old. The new instructions would be something like, "I am lovable, I am enough, I am brave." This type of session could be repeated more than once. Hypnosis is valuable. It allows you to access and heal a part of your mind that you may not have conscious memory of.

Exercising is another excellent way to clear stuck energy. You need to get your heart rate up and break a sweat in order to clear stuck energy. I personally like to run, and I know that I've been running long enough because my hands start to sweat. Thirty minutes, for me, is about the right amount of time for this to occur.

I started running at a very low point in my life. For me, when I started, running was definitely a big challenge and something to improve on, and it taught me a lot. I would find myself thinking about quitting almost as soon as I started. I had so many random thoughts that would pop up and try to sabotage my run. But, day by day, I would get through the struggle, and in that process, deeper challenges started to arise. Running made me tougher mentally. It was something I didn't love, but it was something that helped me heal.

Knowing about the chakras, I was drawn to yoga. My little town of 5,000 people has a yoga studio, Still Water Yoga, that is amazing. The class that resonated with me was the Vinyasa Flow. There are times when I found yoga to be difficult, but I knew it too was helping me heal. It seems that often the emphasis of the sessions matched perfectly with what I needed at the time.

I often went to the chiropractor when I was working forty-plus hours a week at the pharmacy. Standing on the hard floor all day with no breaks is difficult on the body. Holding a phone in the crook of the neck is not helpful either. I didn't realize how effective the chiropractic adjustments were until I didn't need them anymore. I would go get the adjustment and then go back into the environment that created the issues that created my need for the adjustment—it was a vicious cycle. Now that I am not working all of those hours at the pharmacy, I don't need to go to the chiropractor!

EMDR therapy is also an effective way to clear trauma. In my journey to heal my energy, I started seeing a therapist who specialized in child abuse. The sessions I had with her were difficult, as most therapy is. On one hand, I was gaining clarity on my childhood and learning about my fears; I had so many. But on the other hand, I felt raw and exposed. I wasn't feeling better; I felt like I was getting worse.

I decided to see a psychic. I wanted to speak with someone who spoke the same language as I did and could shed some light on what I was going through. I wanted her to tell me what I could do to get better, to feel better. I was dying on the inside.

I met with Angela Pennisi, a psychic medium. I told her I was in therapy and I felt like it was making me worse. I was feeling very conflicted. "Please help me," I said.

Angela told me I was getting the wrong kind of therapy. She told me I should do something different, something out-of-the-box and away from home. Interestingly enough, my sister, who lived in Portland, Oregon, was trying to get me to come visit to see someone she knew and trusted. So, I flew out to Portland and spent a few days with family and a few intensive days with a wonderful lady named Diane Ulicsni, who introduced me to EMDR therapy. She explained to me that I had trauma stuck in my brain and the talk therapy I was doing was basically making it worse. I needed to release the stuck trauma. The EMDR therapy was what helped me heal, but as with all healings, it happened in layers.

Angela also gave me one other piece of advice: She told me that I needed to get back to work. At this stage, I was not working at the pharmacy and my healing work came to a complete halt during my healing crisis. After my trip to Portland, I was feeling better and I was ready to get back to work. Angela offered her office space to me to hold a group energy healing, and that was the start of something new for me.

During this time, I also discovered that I love to paint. This was something new for me because although I don't remember ever being artistic, I found it therapeutic and it helped me reconnect with my inner being, my soul self. I lost that connection going back to my NDE. I didn't know who I was, and I was trying to find my way back home. I was trying to reconnect with my true self and painting helped me do that. I started to trust myself again and listened to my intuition about what I needed to do to help myself heal. Painting or doing other creative projects won't clear stuck energy, but it will help connect to your true self and be confident in being able to guide yourself.

Months later, my healing journey took me down the rabbit hole once again and pushed me straight back into therapy. This time, my husband dragged me to a new therapist in the area who specialized in EMDR therapy. This would be round three for me. I wasn't excited about the process, and this time, I had an audience. My husband sat in on all of the sessions except the last one I went to. It all ended very strangely. At the end of my session, the therapist didn't reach for her calendar to schedule an appointment. She walked me to the door and said that I didn't need to come back. She told me that I didn't need her anymore, but if I did, to call and make an appointment. It was the strangest thing. My therapist fired me.

My family encouraged me to find another therapist, but I felt a sense of calm and decided to follow my own guidance. My own guidance told me that I needed to go it alone. I needed to do this for myself, by myself. It wasn't a popular decision.

Intuitive energy healing is what I do for others in order to help them heal. I sense what is stuck in my clients' energetic fields and I channel energy to clear it. The energy I use is that of the angels. After my NDE, I lost my connection to angels for most of my adult life. I didn't remember them or anything about my connection to them. During my healing process, I started having visions of a group of angels. I started painting the angels and the images I kept seeing in my mind. I wondered what they were trying to tell me. In my NDE, I died and stood in a circle of angels. They told me that I had to go back. I didn't do what I came to Earth to do, and I wouldn't remember them until the time was right. My soul was begging me to remember. My intuition, that voice I heard, was nudging me along.

Of course, there are other types of energy healers out there, such as Reiki and Chios. While these do not personally resonate with me, you need to work with a healer and method that resonates with you.

You're probably wondering, "Where should I start?" If you have trauma in your background, I would suggest EMDR therapy or RTT hypnotherapy to begin with. Having a someone to talk to about your trauma is essential. Your friends and family get tired of hearing about it, and this often chases people away. Having said that, not all therapists are created equal. You may need to shop around.

If you're like me and you have no idea that your past is rifled with trauma, then you need to see someone like myself, a healer. Also, if you were working on healing for years and you just haven't quite figured out what is at the core of your issues, call me. You don't have to spin your wheels for a long period of time. Find someone to help you.

How Do I Know If I Have Stuck Energy?

"There are no limitations to the self except that you believe in."

– Anonymous

Knowing the telltale signs of stuck energy will teach you to manage your own energy and stop looking outside yourself for the answers. We all look to others when something is ailing us. Mostly, as a society, we seek medical attention to solve our physical problems. We want an answer now, and the solution to that problem, for many, is to take a pill. Taking pills in our society is synonymous with, "I don't have to take responsibility for what is happening here."

The body's sickness/disease is one of the final places that stuck energy shows up. This energy moved from the emotional, the mental, and the soul body before it ever showed up in the physical body. The energy made all sorts of attempts to get your attention in many ways. Those attempts could be physical aches and pains, anxiety, dreams, depression, or any ailment that affects the body, mind, or soul.

For example, you may be stuck in some area of your life— perhaps relationships are a struggle. You could be involved in risky behaviors. You may have difficulty keeping a job. There is a recurring pattern in your life that is showing you something that needs to be healed.

For me, that pattern of reoccurrence told me that I was in the wrong career. I thought if I had the right career, the sick feeling I had would magically disappear. I knew intuitively that something in my life was off, that there was something wrong with me, but I dare not speak about it. Instead of examining those feelings more deeply, I continued to look outside myself to solve what needed to be healed on the inside. I didn't remember the trauma I had. My brain did an amazing job of trying to keep me safe. The mind will do everything possible to keep you safe, and in doing so, you may not be able to heal.

Anger is another sign of internal strife but realize that anger is really a cover emotion for something much deeper inside. When you feel angry, ask what this is really about. Typically, the answer is a fear you have or hurt feelings.

Being triggered is another sign that something needs to be healed. I once met a woman who was a friend of a friend. Although I didn't know her, I instantly did not like her. She triggered me, even though I had no reason not to like her. It took me some time and some healing to realize that she was just like my mother and that was why she was triggering me. When you are triggered by something or someone, it's just an opportunity to see what needs to be healed. This isn't a reflection of them; it's a reflection of you.

Emotions are often high when there is something that needs to be healed. I hear people say, "I have so much anxiety," or, "I'm so depressed." These are symptoms of a deeper issue. Unfortunately, most of the time, when someone starts experiencing these feelings, they look outside themselves to self-soothe with drugs, alcohol, or through medicating with prescription drugs.

Insomnia is another sign that you have an energy issue somewhere. Although we all have times when sleep is disrupted, I'm not talking about those experiences. Rather, I am speaking directly to those who don't sleep without assistance of drugs or alcohol. There is something in the mind that haunts that person, whether consciously or not.

Over the years, I had a few people who came back to me time and time again. When they were being triggered or stuck in a life situation, they trusted me to show them what was wanting to be healed rather than ignored.

These are a few signs that you have stuck energy, and I've given you a few examples of how this works so you can see or relate the material to your own life.

I could have benefited deeply by utilizing a counselor in my twenties, when the dissatisfaction in my work first cropped up, but it never occurred to me. I simply thought I chose the wrong career. I would suggest counseling to anyone who may feel that something is "off." From a personal standpoint, it's beneficial to have someone to talk to who doesn't have a vested interest in your story.

The Soul Chakra

*"If you don't believe in miracles,
perhaps you've forgotten you are one."*

– Anonymous

I spent years developing my intuitive healing modality. Literally overnight, everything changed when I was introduced to the soul chakra, also called the zero chakra. I discovered this chakra literally by accident (and I don't believe in accidents). In the middle of the night, the phone began ringing, and while I was trying to get to it, I missed a step, or three. I heard a crack and I went down.

I knew all the right things to do to heal my foot. I probably should have gone to the emergency room, because I was pretty sure it was broken. However, it was a weekend and I decided that if my foot wasn't any better the next day, I would go to the doctor. I spent the day on the couch. I wrapped the foot, iced it, and kept it elevated. The following day, my foot was better, but I realized it was going to take some time to heal. I got the crutches out and babied the foot for a while. There's no way I was going to the doctor to have him tell me what I already knew.

I had a sense of calm about my foot and after a few days, I started to wonder what this experience was trying to teach me. The crack that I heard was my soul cracking open, not literally but metaphorically. I didn't need a doctor to help me heal, but my recovery was going to take some time. I already healed other aspects of my life—the emotional and mental fields. It was time to take care of my soul.

This was to be the final phase of healing for me, and oddly enough, the part that was missing in my energy work—the part that would turn my work upside down.

Clearing the soul chakra is the most important part of an energy healing because it is the place or the origin of sickness and disease. When the source of sickness is removed, the body is able to do its amazing work healing itself.

A wound to the soul can occur any time after a soul enters the body, beginning shortly after conception (seven to eight weeks in-utero) and up until an individual's late twenties. The brain is not developed until almost thirty years old and is therefore susceptible to a wound. Anybody in this age bracket cannot process traumatic events, while someone over the age of thirty is more equipped to process trauma simply because the brain is fully developed.

If trauma is not processed, it remains in the subconscious mind. This trauma is like a computer program that runs in the background of everything you do until you do something to change it.

In my experience, five percent of my clients had soul issues that occurred in-utero, as they picked up emotions/feelings from their mother of not being wanted or even loved. Eighty-five percent of my clients had some sort of trauma before the age of nine, and ten percent of my clients were in their teens to late twenties when their trauma occurred.

Clearly, wounding your soul in-utero would be the most difficult to discover unless you were told that your mother had a difficult or unwanted pregnancy. In-utero, a child's brain is just forming, and his or her sense of well-being is absorbed through the mother. Negative feelings are clearly felt, wounding a child.

The larger group of kids aged nine and under don't often remember their trauma because their brains are not fully developed. At this age, information is flowing directly into the subconscious mind, and soon the partition between the conscious and subconscious mind will form.

The older kids/young adults experience their trauma a little later in life. Still unable to process their trauma, older children and teens often resort to drugs and alcohol to cope with their anxieties. These kids often know exactly what caused their trauma and will tell you that they have PTSD or other types of distress.

Remember how my foot was injured, and how I knew this was a soul issue? A person who has an issue with their soul chakra will typically have issues with their feet because the left foot is more internal and represents the soul itself, while the right foot is the expression of the soul into the physical world.

Meet Susan

Susan came to me when she was struggling in a relationship. For her, the story was always the same. Relationships didn't end well because the men in her life always left her.

In a soul healing, I found that her mother did not want to have another baby. Susan's mother already had two children when she became pregnant, and both children were both under four-years-old. Susan's mother tried to take the matter into her own hands and force a miscarriage by throwing herself down the stairs. She couldn't have another baby, and thought, "Who will take care of me?"

Susan obviously did not die but never felt loved by her mother, and her twin sister was stillborn.

For Susan, feeling unloved and abandoned were a few themes that played out for her over and over in her life.

Meet Ann

Ann came to see me before a scheduled surgery and informed me that she had uterine cancer and she wanted to do whatever she could to heal quickly and easily. I found a victimization wound within Ann, and she told me that she was date raped and became pregnant. Her mother forced her into marriage to the man that raped her. Ann lost her baby, but since then had other children. She long since forgave her husband. This victimization trauma was not the source of Ann's cancer as one might think but rather the unresolved issue with her mother. This trauma directly imposed by her mother was the source of the cancer.

Following Ann's surgery, she told me the tumor was removed and did not spread. There was no further treatment and Ann is free of sickness today.

The Original Wound

"It always seems impossible until it is done."

– Anonymous

Located within the soul chakra is what I call the original wound. This is the root or foundation of all sickness/disease. It is also the wound that needs to be healed. In my work over the years, I healed from the outside in. It was effective, and all I knew at the time was that I would address what was coming up on the outside or what issues were on the surface. My healing was much the same—I was healing the next trauma that was emerging. What I came to discover was that there is an original wound that is at the root of it all.

The original wound is always attached to the soul. People are always seeking to heal this wound even if it is on the subconscious level. A person may be seeking medical attention, or they were like me and were looking outside themselves to fix or heal something that they were feeling on the inside. More likely than not, they are self-medicating.

Think of the wound as the roots of a tree. Without those roots, the tree cannot stand. If you keep cutting the branches and never get to the roots, the tree will grow back. This is the reason why people don't recover from sickness or disease—they haven't healed the original wound, the wound at the soul level. This also makes me think of people who were in therapy for thirty years. I'm not knocking therapy; I'm just wondering how effective it is if someone still goes back for thirty years. My point is, after all that time in therapy, why aren't they healed?

My mother and mother-in-law both died from breast cancer. It's an ugly disease. My mother-in-law's cancer was very aggressive. She had chemo, radiation, and surgery, and at one point I remember doctors declared her cancer-free—but that was all a lie. Within a short while, the cancer returned more aggressive than ever and spread to other areas. The cancer was treated physically, and the doctors would tell us that they didn't know how it started or where it came from. All the doctors did know was how to attack what they saw physically. What they didn't see was the original wound, or the cause that created that mess of cancer.

Sadly, I wasn't aware of my spiritual gifts when my mother-in-law was sick, and I wish I could have helped her. I don't know what her original wound was, but I'm certain it had to do with being and feeling loved, because breast cancer is directedly related to the heart chakra and those feelings.

Shortly after my mother-in-law died, my mother was diagnosed with a different type of breast cancer. Less than four months after my mother's diagnosis, she died. My mother had very little treatment because by the time she was diagnosed, the cancer ravaged her body.

My mother discovered a lump in her breast the week I was married. She said she didn't want to ruin my wedding by announcing this news. It would be sixteen years later before she went to the doctor. In fact, it was other symptoms of leg and knee pain that sent her for medical attention. By this time, the cancer progressed, and it was too late.

Still, at this time, I didn't discover that I was a healer and never heard about such things. I would have helped her if I knew. Following my mother's death, she started visiting me in my dreams. Over the next few years, she would spill the beans on my childhood trauma that I couldn't remember, and on her childhood as well.

My mother told me that she was sexually abused by her father starting at the age of six. She had a child by her father as a very young age and gave that child up for adoption. My mother's original wound stems from that violation. Her heart chakra was closed off, she didn't feel loved, and she gave away a part of herself. She never healed from that.

The original wound is the cause of all sickness. If the original wound is healed, the physical body will heal. The tricky part is finding that wound. For some, the wound is buried deep in the subconscious. For others, they may not have heard of this type of healing work. It's not on their radar.

Meet Michelle

Michelle's original wound begins at birth when she and her mother almost died. The doctor told her father that they could only save one of them and that he would have to choose. Michelle's father chose her, and after that decision, he went to his vehicle and gathered his shotgun. He arrived back to the hospital and informed the doctor and the staff that he better save both of them or he will die.

Both Michelle and her mother survived, but there was a deep resentment towards Michelle due to the choice her father made. This was the start of years of abuse and torment by her mother.

One might think the original wound would be the abuse by her mother, but her wound began at birth when her father chose her. Michelle felt the pain and anguish that her mother felt of not being chosen. She felt the rejection and has throughout her life.

Meet Dee

Dee found herself not feeling loved. She sought a great deal of self-help through various coaching programs but found herself right back to where she started: not feeling loved. Intellectually, she knew this wasn't true. She had loving parents and siblings. She had a significant other but wasn't convinced he was the one.

Dee's original wound originated in-utero. Her mother had a late pregnancy as she was in her mid-40s when she was conceived. There was an instance when Dee's mother realized that she was pregnant and was less than thrilled. Dee's parents adored her, but the negative feelings that Dee's mother felt initially stuck to Dee like glue. These were the feelings that Dee wasn't able to escape.

My original wound took years to find. You heard the saying, "You don't know what you don't know." I didn't know that my childhood was rifled with abuse. Each phase (there were several) took my healing to a deeper level. Each time that I would get new insights and heal one aspect, I would think, "Finally, it's over." But more would come. I was peeling back each layer, piece by piece. It was a daunting task, but necessary in order to fully understand my healing work and to heal myself.

Early in my healing and discovery, I asked my mother to leave me and my family alone. She left as I requested. I didn't hear from her. However, I did continue to receive messages, dreams, and visions about my childhood. I knew I was a medium but didn't question who I was talking to. It was my spirit guide; I knew that much. The messages I received came from a familiar voice I often heard throughout my life. I heard that voice when I met my husband for the first time, telling me that Steve would be my husband. I trusted that voice. The voice didn't lie, and it proved to be true over and over. But that's all I knew. I didn't know anything else about it.

As I entered the final phase of my healing—that of the soul chakra and the original wound—I started having visions of a girl.

> *Vision: In front of me was an oversized white wooden door. I opened the door, and peeked down the long hallway. There stood a beautiful young girl with long dark hair. She was wearing a long, blue, sparkly gown that hugged her body. She walked toward me and placed her hands up in front of my own. I felt the energy pulsate between our palms. I began to cry.*

Over and over I had this vision. Like a dream, the vision repeated until the message was understood. I didn't know who she was. I didn't know what she wanted or what her personal connection to me was. I started to paint her and thought that may help me get in touch with her. I didn't realize that she was my spirit guide, helping me to heal.

Healing the original wound took some time. As it was revealed to me, I finally understood the vision I was having and was able to heal my childhood in totality. In order for me to be completely healed, I had to heal my original wound. It was nothing that I was looking for or expected.

When my mother became pregnant with me, she didn't know who my father was. She was still being abused by her father. She took matters into her own hands and tried to end her pregnancy. She thought she ended it, but there were two babies—twins. I had a twin sister, and while my sister died, I lived. My twin sister is the one who speaks to me. It's her voice I heard throughout my life; she was the one guiding me. Losing her, and the fashion in which it happened, was the source of my original wound.

I share this with you so that you know it is possible to discover and heal your own original wound. It may not be as dramatic as my own story, but if you have sickness/disease in your life, you have something to heal. This discovery flipped my work inside-out. I no longer heal others from the outside-in, but go right to the original wound, since it is the foundation of all other energetic blocks. Finally, we can stop peeling back the layers by healing one thing at a time by uncovering the original wound.

Please Help Me Eliminate This Stuck Energy

"Quiet the mind and the soul will speak."

– Buddha

Healing your chakras and the original wound is something that everyone can do for themselves. I gave you some guidelines of what needs to be done, as well as different ways to clear the negative energy. You can definitely do this by yourself; I did it, and you can too.

However, there is one major downside to healing on your own—it takes years. I was working on healing myself for close to five years. Truth is, I started searching when I graduated from college. I just didn't realize this on a conscious level.

You can wait until you have a full-blown illness before you look for your original wound, or you can be proactive and take care of it now.

The number one thing that everybody should do is develop their innate gifts, their intuition. Everybody has intuition, and as you work with it, it will expand. You need to know exactly how your intuition speaks to you. Pay close attention to your dream time. Everybody has their own dream style, and once you understand what your style is, you will open the door to valuable insight from the spirit world. Dreams are a high level of intuition.

Intuition is a valuable asset to your physical existence, as it will guide you along the way as it has for me. I created several e-courses about intuition, dreams, and energy healing, and while you heal your wound, I would go through them in that order, because that is how this program was designed.

The energy healing course I offer online is the companion course to this book, including various methods of healing that I go over in videos and in reading. I also share intuitive energy healing, as that's my specialty. After that, I review the chakras in detail, giving you an idea of what chakra issue you are experiencing based on the illness or symptoms you may be experiencing. As you learned, the energy centers correspond with various parts of the body. The course will take you through the causes of stuck energy: emotions, feelings, beliefs, and trauma. I will teach you ways to clear the stuck energy through tools that I utilized in my personal healing. I know these tools are effective, but they take time. As discussed here, the course will answer the important question, "How do I know if I have stuck energy?"

As I experienced, energy healing by yourself takes a long time. I often wondered, if I healed all at once, what would that look like? Would I know everything I know now, or would I have missed the opportunity to learn the truth about my life?

Healing layer-by-layer is a slow process, and most people won't take the time, not because they don't want to but because they don't know what needs to be done.

Here are the crucial steps to healing each layer and recovering from your original wound:

1. Identify the problem.
2. Establish a plan. If your plan doesn't work, adjust the plan or seek guidance.
3. Get to a therapist or find a healer.

4. Call me and set up an appointment.
5. Be patient with yourself.

I also created several guided meditations to assist you in your intuition development. The most sought-after meditation is entitled, "Come Sit by Me." This meditation was designed to help you, the listener, connect with loved ones in your dream time, also called a dream visitation. You don't have to be a medium in order to connect with spirits in your dream time. If you are a medium (lucky you, that's a gift), you are able to connect during your awake time as well, but everybody can have a dream visitation, and this can help you on your journey to heal your trauma.

All Sickness Is Stuck Energy

"Energy speaks louder than words."

– Anonymous

There is no difference between stuck energy and sickness. Sickness is the result of stuck energy or an energetic block. However, not all stuck energy is sickness.

Energy is a vibration, and high-vibrating, positive energy is not the problem; lower-vibration energy of a negative nature becomes stuck energy. Left alone long enough, stuck energy will eventually migrate to the body and become sickness/disease.

To help you in your journey towards healing, here is a list of energies that lower a person's vibration, as well as positive energy/high vibration.

Low Vibration Energy
- Emotional pain
- Heartache
- Doubt
- Worry
- Trauma
- Gossip
- Spite
- Fear

- Toxic people
- Regret
- Jealousy
- Insecurity
- Shame

High Vibration Energy

- Joy
- Happiness
- Love
- Gratitude
- Amusement
- Hope
- Pride
- Serenity
- Calmness
- Abundance
- Bravery
- Acceptance
- Accomplishment
- Humor

Fill your life with positive vibrational energy and eliminate the negative vibrational energy if possible. If eliminating negative energy is not possible, limit your exposure to such energy.

It's so important to develop your intuition in order to strengthen the voice of your soul. Listen for the clues that something is off. You should be able to feel something being off, but you won't feel this if you don't have a strong connection to your soul.

Take care of your physical body. It is not replaceable, and it is the home of your soul. Make sure that you eat good food, drink pure water, eliminate toxins whenever possible, rest, and exercise. Your body will thank you. The importance of eating mostly healthy foods cannot be overstated here, because the body needs nutrients in order to maintain a healthy state. Our diets became inundated with processed food, which lack nutrition and contain so much sugar that we become addicted to bad food.

As you recall what you learned in this book, think back to the chakras and how stuck energy here ultimately causes physical harm to the body. You know different ways of clearing stuck energy for yourself and who to call if you need assistance. You are now aware of what causes stuck energy—feelings, emotions, past life issues, or trauma. This is the tricky part: the mind will try to protect you and keep you safe. It doesn't want you to remember the pain or heartache. Remember also that children cannot process trauma and our brains are not fully developed until our late twenties. You may need assistance processing trauma whether you realize it or not.

Healing is not a race, it's a marathon. It takes time to peel back the layers and layers that become stuck in an energetic field. In traditional medicine, physicians treat the physical body only. In energy healing, the mind, emotions, and the soul are also treated. Just because you can't see something doesn't mean it isn't there. No one questions whether or not a person has a soul. Of course, we have a soul; we just can't see it. The same is true for the other energetic bodies and the chakras. We must treat the whole body, mind, and soul.

You learned how to recognize if you have stuck energy. Stuck energy appears in various forms other than sickness. You may be stuck in an area of life, unable to get past a problem. You may have a reoccurring pattern, such as bad relationships, risky behaviors, or inability to keep a job. There is some area in your life that you feel unfulfilled. These are clues that something is blocked for you. We also discussed triggers and how a trigger appears to show you a place in your life that needs to be healed. The trigger isn't about someone else; it's about you.

I introduced you to the soul chakra, also called the zero chakra, where the original wound resides. This needs to be healed in order for physical sickness to be healed. The original wound can be formed anytime, starting in-utero until a person's late twenties. Most people won't remember the childhood wound, as their mind buried it. Time won't heal this wound. It takes deep, inner work. You can heal it by yourself or seek professional help.

It's not necessary to peel back the layers as I did over the years. I learned that if you go straight to the original wound and pull it out, the rest of the layers of hurt and trauma fall apart as well. A tree isn't able to stand without roots, and the roots are the original wound. The tree is the sickness and various energetic blocks that grow from those roots. In my own healing work, I was merely trimming the tree. Eliminating the original wound is what freed me.

In order for our medical system to change, we have to change.

> *"No problem can be solved from the level of*
> *consciousness that it was created."*
>
> – Albert Einstein

The problem is how we manage sickness. We, as a society, have it all wrong. We are looking with our physical eyes to see the unseen. We are using our logical minds rather than our intuition to recognize what needs addressing. We must turn, look deep inside, and listen to the language of our soul.

Modern medicine placed its practices inside the box of mainstream, societal norms. Any method of healing that doesn't fit in that box is not considered. These practices are often ridiculed, mocked, and devalued. If insurance doesn't pay for a service, people don't want it, thinking that because insurance doesn't pay for a service, it must not have value. We let an entire industry manipulate us into believing that modern medicine is the only way. We've been following the leader, and the leader is lost. It's time for a shift.

There seems to be a complete loss of personal responsibility. When given the option to modify a behavior, such as weight, in order to lower blood pressure or to change diet in order to modify cholesterol, the patient would rather take a pill. Take control of your life. Don't neglect it now and work on it later. Your body houses your soul and it needs to be cared for.

Stop looking outside yourself to heal, because healing is an inside job.

Acknowledgments

*"To be yourself in a world that is constantly
trying to make you something else
is the greatest accomplishment."*

– Ralph Waldo Emerson

I breathe a sigh of relief as I write this final piece. I was writing this book for ten years.

The book wasn't always about energy healing; it actually started out about my girls and how I opened up to my gifts when they were little. They were my teachers. I was circling around this topic for years, seeking truth and clarity.

Healing is my art, and I am thrilled to finally be able to share it with you. This is my soul's mission to help change the world, to help heal the world. My wish for you is that you are able to heal your soul and be who you are meant to be.

My story is not a pretty one. I shared what I needed to share in order to explain my work in detail. The rest of the story, I will share at a later time.

I am thankful for those that helped me through my healing process and writing this book.

Thank you to Angela Lauria and The Author Incubator's team, as well as to Jesse Krieger and the Lifestyle Entrepreneurs Press Publishing team for helping me bring this book to print.

Thank You

Thank you for reading *Is This Sickness or an Energy Block?: Know the Difference and What to Do About It.*

I hope you are well on your way to healing.

Visit amykeast.com for up-to-date information on where I will be appearing or if you would like to schedule your private session.

Join me on Instagram! Tag me in a post with you and your book: @amykeast, #soulsurge. I would also like to invite you to join me on Facebook at

https://www.facebook.com/amykeastintuitive/ or join my private Facebook group by searching the "Groups" section of Facebook: Spirit Signs by Amy Keast.

About the Author

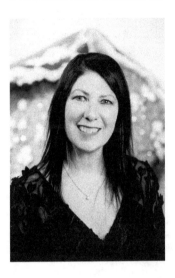

Amy Keast, author of *Is This Sickness or an Energy Block?: Know the Difference and What to Do About It,* is a pharmacist-turned-Intuitive Energy Healer—a soul healer. Having a near death experience when she was eight years old, Amy lost her spiritual gifts and sense of who she really was. Amy's spiritual gifts and true self reemerged, and in the process, she created her own healing modality.

Working in the medical field as a pharmacist for most of her adult life, Amy has a unique perspective about how our society is dealing with sickness/disease. She flipped the dynamic from looking outside ourselves to looking within in order to heal. Amy uses her intuition to identify stuck energy in a person's energetic field. She then channels spirit energy to clear that stuck energy. In addition to offering private and group energy sessions,

Amy is a public speaker sharing her unique perspective on healing. Amy also offers e-courses to enhance your own intuition, learn more about your dreams, or expand your knowledge of energy healing. She is the creator of Soul Surge, which includes the courses Intuition 101, Dreams 101, and Energy Healing 101.

Amy is married with two adult children (Madison and Ellen) and lives in Harlan, Iowa, with her husband Steve and their long-haired dachshund Paul.